MEDICAL ETHICS COOKBOOK

Enjoy fast and easy complete delicious friendly recipes to Nourish your health from Ethics pain plus 30day meal plan to stay Longlife.

JENNIFER .S COLE

Copyright © 2024 JENNIFER .S COLE
Allright Reserved

No part of this publication may be reproduced or transmitted in any form or by any means, electronically or mechanically, including photocopying, recording or any information storage or retrieved system, without the prior permission in writing from the copyright owner.

TABLE OF CONTENT

INTRODUCTION... 6
Chapter 1:DEFINITION OF MEDICAL ETHICS............ 9
Chapter 2:MEDICAL ETHICS' ADVANTAGES........... 12
Chapter 3: COOKING IN ACCORDANCE WITH
MEDICAL ETHICS.. 16
Chapter 4:BREAKFAST RECIPES........................... 21
Recipe 1: Autonomy Omelette................................ 21
Recipe 2: Beneficence Smoothie............................ 23
Recipe 3: Non-maleficence Pancakes..................... 25
Recipe 4: Justice Parfait.. 27
Recipe 5: Confidentiality Cereal Bowl..................... 28
Recipe 6: Integrity Frittata..................................... 30
Recipe 7: Compassionate Breakfast Burrito........... 32
Recipe 8: Dignity French Toast.............................. 34
Recipe 9: Confidentiality Yogurt Bowl.....................35
Recipe 10: Advocacy Avocado Toast...................... 37
Chapter 5: LUNCH RECIPES................................... 39
Recipe 1: Informed Consent Salad......................... 39
Recipe 2: Beneficence Buddha Bowl...................... 41
Recipe 3: Non-maleficence Veggie Wrap................ 43
Recipe 4: Justice Grain Bowl................................. 45
Recipe 5: Confidentiality Chicken Salad................. 47
Recipe 6: Respect Stir-Fry.....................................49
Recipe 7: Compassion Lentil Soup......................... 52
Recipe 8: Integrity Quinoa Salad........................... 54
Recipe 9: Advocacy Veggie Sandwich..................... 56
Recipe 10: Trust Tacos...58

Chapter 6: DINNER RECIPES 60
Recipe 1: Autonomy Stir-Fry 60
Recipe 2: Beneficence Baked Salmon 62
Recipe 3: Non-maleficence Veggie Pasta 65
Recipe 4: Justice Stuffed Peppers 67
Recipe 5: Confidentiality Chicken Enchiladas 69
Recipe 6: Fidelity Meatloaf 71
Recipe 7: Non-maleficence Mushroom Risotto 74
Recipe 8: Veracity Vegetable Lasagna 76
Recipe 9: Dignity Roast Chicken 79
Recipe 10: Accountability Stuffed Eggplant 81
Chapter 7: SNACKS RECIPES 84
Recipe 1: Autonomy Energy Bites 84
Recipe 2: Beneficence Fruit and Nut Mix 86
Recipe 3: Non-maleficence Veggie Sticks with Hummus 88
Recipe 4: Justice Apple Slices with Almond Butter 89
Recipe 5: Confidentiality Greek Yogurt Parfait 91
Recipe 6: Integrity Granola Bars 92
Recipe 7: Compassionate Caprese Skewers 94
Recipe 8: Respectful Rice Cakes 96
Recipe 9: Justice Trail Mix 97
Recipe 10: Confidentiality Yogurt Dip with Veggies 99
Chapter 8: DESSERT RECIPES 100
Recipe 1: Autonomy Apple Crisp 101
Recipe 2: Beneficence Berry Parfait 103
Recipe 3: Non-maleficence Chocolate Avocado Mousse 104
Recipe 4: Justice Fruit Salad 106

Recipe 5: Fidelity Peanut Butter Cookies............... 108
Recipe 6: Respectful Raspberry Sorbet................. 110
Recipe 7: Integrity Chocolate Bark........................ 112
Recipe 8: Compassionate Carrot Cake Muffins..... 114
Recipe 9: Justice Lemon Bars................................116
Recipe 10: Fidelity Pecan Pie Bites........................ 119
Chapter 9:APPETIZERS AND HEALTHY RECIPES 121
Recipe 1: Empowerment Veggie Dip...................... 121
Recipe 2: Non-maleficence Hummus Platter......... 122
Recipe 3: Beneficence Quinoa Salad Cups........... 124
Recipe 4: Justice Stuffed Mushrooms................... 126
Recipe 5: Confidentiality Cucumber Roll-Ups....... 129
Recipe 6: Empathy Edamame Salad....................... 131
Recipe 7: Integrity Stuffed Bell Peppers................ 133
Recipe 8: Non-maleficence Fruit Salsa with Cinnamon Chips.. 136
Recipe 9: Justice Greek Stuffed Mushrooms........ 138
Recipe 10: Confidentiality Caprese Skewers......... 140
30DAY MEAL PLAN.. 142
Day 1:..142
Day 2:..142
Day 3:..142
Day 4:..143
Day 5:..143
Day 6:..144
Day 7:..144
Day 8:..145
Day 9:..145
Day 10:..145

Day 11: 146
Day 12: 146
Day 13: 147
Day 14: 147
Day 15: 148
Day 16: 148
Day 17: 149
Day 18: 149
Day 19: 150
Day 20: 150
Day 21: 151
Day 22: 151
Day 23: 152
Day 24: 152
Day 25: 152
Day 26: 153
Day 27: 153
Day 28: 154
Day 29: 154
Day 30: 155
CONCLUSION.. 155
THE END..157

INTRODUCTION

"Welcome to the Medical Ethics Cookbook, where compassion meets cuisine and nourishment meets noble purpose.

As healthcare professionals, we've seen firsthand the impact that food can have on our patients' lives. We've witnessed the healing power of a warm meal, the comfort of a familiar flavor, and the joy of sharing a meal with loved ones. But we've also seen the devastating effects of poor nutrition, the confusion of conflicting dietary advice, and the struggle to prioritize self-care in a demanding profession.

That's why we created this cookbook - to bring together the wisdom of medical ethics and the warmth of good food. Within these pages, you'll find:

- Delicious, easy-to-make recipes that prioritize whole, nutritious ingredients

- Inspiring stories of healthcare professionals who embody the principles of medical ethics
- Practical tips for navigating the complex landscape of healthcare and nutrition

This cookbook is more than just a collection of recipes - it's a testament to the power of food to heal, connect, and inspire. It's a reminder that, as healthcare professionals, we have the privilege and responsibility to nourish not just our patients' bodies, but their spirits as well.

Join us on this culinary journey, and discover the transformative power of food, compassion, and community. Let's cook, let's care, and let's inspire a healthier, more compassionate world - one delicious bite at a time!"

Chapter 1: DEFINITION OF MEDICAL ETHICS

The beliefs and tenets that direct the practice of medicine are the subject of the field of medical ethics. In order to protect patients' rights and dignity and to build confidence between patients and healthcare professionals, it entails applying moral concepts to medical decisions. End-of-life care, informed consent, patient confidentiality, and the allocation of limited medical resources are just a few of the many topics covered by medical ethics.

Among the fundamentals of medical ethics are:

Autonomy: Honoring the patient's prerogative to choose their own medical providers. This entails making certain that patients are properly informed about the risks and advantages of each treatment option.

Beneficence: The duty of healthcare professionals to behave in the patient's best interest by fostering their wellbeing and carrying out beneficial actions for them.

Principle of non-maleficence: "Do no harm." Whenever feasible, healthcare professionals should try to reduce risks and refrain from hurting their patients.

Justice is ensuring that medical resources and treatments are distributed fairly and that no one is discriminated against while making decisions.

In addition, medical ethics include tackling more complicated problems like:

Preserving patient data's privacy is known as confidentiality.
Ensuring that patients are aware of the nature of their treatment and willingly consent to it is known as informed consent.

Making decisions on advanced directives, euthanasia, and palliative care at the end of life.

Allocating resources fairly involves deciding how to divide up the few available medical resources, such as transplantable organs or access to experimental therapies.

Research ethics: Ensuring the moral conduct of medical research while safeguarding the welfare and rights of participants.

Legal frameworks that differ by nation and area and professional standards of conduct, such those offered by the American Medical Association (AMA), serve as guidelines for medical ethics. In order to ensure that the treatment they offer is both morally and practically sound, these recommendations assist healthcare professionals in navigating the ethical conundrums that arise in clinical practice and research.

Chapter 2: MEDICAL ETHICS' ADVANTAGES

Medical ethics creates a framework for moral decision-making and promotes integrity and trust in the healthcare system, which benefits patients and healthcare practitioners alike. Here are a few of the main advantages:

Increases Patient Trust: Patients and healthcare professionals can develop trust by abiding by ethical standards like autonomy, informed consent, and confidentiality. When patients feel valued and understood, they are more inclined to comply with treatment plans and disclose sensitive information.

Enhances Patient Care: By adhering to ethical standards, patients are guaranteed to receive care that is optimal for them. Better health results result from healthcare providers prioritizing patient well-being and minimizing harm, guided by principles such as beneficence and non-maleficence.

Encourages Justice and Fairness: Ethical principles guarantee the equitable and fair distribution of healthcare resources. This aids in the equitable distribution of resources, such as access to experimental medicines or organs for transplantation, and the selection of patients who get care.

Supports Professional Integrity: By establishing unambiguous guidelines for conduct, medical ethics protect the integrity of the medical field. This promotes healthcare providers' continued high standards of responsibility and professionalism.

Directs Decision-Making: Ethical principles offer a methodical approach to decision-making in difficult circumstances with moral quandaries. This aids medical professionals in resolving difficult issues including conflicts of interest, patient treatment rejection, and end-of-life care.

Protects Patient Rights: Ethical norms make ensuring that patients' rights are upheld, including their right to privacy, their ability to make educated decisions about their own health, and their right to courteous, nondiscriminatory treatment.

Improves Communication: Transparency and honesty are ensured by clear ethical rules, which facilitate communication between patients and healthcare practitioners. This promotes improved communication and teamwork during the therapeutic process.

Promotes Continuous Improvement: Healthcare professionals are encouraged to participate in ongoing education and development by ethical values. Maintaining current knowledge of medical advancements and ethical standards is crucial in delivering optimal care.

Avoids Legal Problems: Following moral principles can assist in avoiding legal problems with malpractice or patient rights violations. It offers a foundation of protection that complies with rules and regulations.

Encourages a Positive Work Environment: Ethical behavior helps to create a helpful and upbeat work atmosphere for healthcare professionals. It encourages cooperation, respect for one another, and a feeling of moral obligation, all of which can lessen burnout and increase job satisfaction.

In the end, medical ethics are crucial to ensure that procedures are carried out fairly, compassionately, and with respect for patients, which benefits both patients and healthcare providers.

Chapter 3: COOKING IN ACCORDANCE WITH MEDICAL ETHICS

An analogy called "cooking with medical ethics" might help explain how medical ethics concepts can be included into healthcare procedures, much like ingredients and recipes are necessary for cooking. The following is an example of how each medical ethics principle could be applied to cooking:

Autonomy (Selecting Your Own Formula):

Healthcare professionals have an obligation to honor patients' autonomy to make decisions about their own care, much as a chef would honor the tastes and choices of the people they provide food for. Making sure patients have access to all the information they need to make well-informed decisions about their treatment options is part of this.

Beneficence (Selecting Healthy Substances):

A chef prepares a dinner that is healthy for the diners by using the greatest and most nutritious ingredients. In a similar vein, healthcare professionals have an obligation to act in their patients' best interests by offering interventions and treatments that advance health and wellbeing.

Non-maleficence (Avoiding Ingredients That Could Hurt):

A chef never uses rotten or dangerous ingredients. In order to reduce risks and prevent injuries, this approach in healthcare encourages providers to refrain from treatments or acts that could hurt patients.

Fair Serving Portions of Justice:

A chef makes sure that each customer receives an equal serving. Justice in healthcare refers to the equitable distribution of medical resources and care, guaranteeing that every patient, regardless of background or circumstances, receives equitable care.

Extra Components in the Cooking Comparison:

Privacy (Redacted Recipes):

Healthcare practitioners are required to protect patient privacy and sensitive information by keeping patient information confidential, much like a chef may withhold some recipes to uphold trust and respect.

Informed Consent (Descriptions of Menu Items):

A menu offers thorough descriptions of every item so that customers may choose their meals with knowledge. In a similar vein, healthcare professionals need to make sure patients are completely aware of all the advantages and disadvantages of each treatment option so they can make an informed choice.

End-of-Life Care: Putting Together a Solace Meal

Caring for someone in distress and preparing a familiar and comforting meal might be compared to compassionate end-of-life care that prioritizes the patient's comfort, dignity, and final wishes.

Allocating Resources (Controlling Ingredients in the Pantry):

A chef needs to stock the pantry carefully and make effective use of the ingredients at hand in order to cook. This translates to prudent medical resource management in the context of healthcare, guaranteeing efficient usage and equitable patient distribution.

Ethics in Research (Recipe Testing):

A chef tests a recipe to make sure it is both tasty and safe to eat before putting it to the menu. Similar to this, medical research needs to be carried out responsibly, taking into account the rights and welfare of participants as well as extensive testing.

By applying this parallel, the difficult concepts of medical ethics are made more approachable and intelligible, underscoring their significance in guaranteeing moral and efficient medical procedures.

Chapter 4: BREAKFAST RECIPES

Recipe 1: Autonomy Omelette

Ingredients:

- 2 large eggs (Patient's choice)
- 1 tablespoon milk (Informed consent)
- 1/4 cup chopped bell peppers (Patient's preferences)
- 1/4 cup chopped onions (Patient's values)

- 1/4 cup shredded cheese (Healthcare provider's guidance)
- Salt and pepper to taste (Respect and understanding)

Instructions:

1. Preparation: Crack the eggs into a bowl and add the milk. Whisk together until well combined, ensuring the patient (eggs) is fully informed and ready for decision-making.
2. Customization: Ask the patient (eggs) about their preferences and add the bell peppers and onions, ensuring their values and choices are respected.
3. Cooking: Heat a non-stick skillet over medium heat and pour in the egg mixture, representing the healthcare provider's guidance and support.

4. Add Cheese: Sprinkle shredded cheese on top, ensuring the patient's choices are well-integrated into the treatment.
5. Season: Add salt and pepper to taste, emphasizing the respect and understanding in the patient-provider relationship.
6. Serve: Fold the omelette and serve hot, celebrating the patient's autonomy in their healthcare decisions.

Recipe 2: Beneficence Smoothie

Ingredients:

- 1 ripe banana (Promoting well-being)
- 1 cup spinach (Health benefits)
- 1/2 cup Greek yogurt (Nutrient-rich)
- 1 cup almond milk (Supporting health)
- 1 tablespoon honey (Sweet care)

- 1/2 cup frozen berries (Additional benefits)

Instructions:

1. Blend Base: Combine the banana and spinach in a blender, focusing on ingredients that promote well-being and health.
2. Add Yogurt: Include Greek yogurt for its nutrient-rich properties, representing actions that benefit the patient.
3. Pour Almond Milk: Add almond milk to support overall health, ensuring the blend is smooth and beneficial.
4. Sweeten: Mix in a tablespoon of honey, adding a touch of care and sweetness to the patient's treatment.
5. Include Berries: Toss in frozen berries for extra health benefits.

6. Serve: Blend until smooth and serve, highlighting the provider's commitment to the patient's well-being.

Recipe 3: Non-maleficence Pancakes

Ingredients:

- 1 cup whole wheat flour (Healthy choices)
- 1 tablespoon baking powder (Safe practices)
- 1 tablespoon sugar (Balanced care)
- 1/4 teaspoon salt (Avoiding harm)
- 1 cup skim milk (Minimizing risks)
- 1 large egg (Patient safety)
- 2 tablespoons vegetable oil (Preventing injury)

Instructions:

1. Mix Dry Ingredients: In a bowl, combine whole wheat flour, baking powder, sugar, and salt, representing the importance of healthy and safe choices.
2. Prepare Wet Ingredients: In another bowl, whisk together skim milk, egg, and vegetable oil, focusing on minimizing risks and ensuring patient safety.
3. Combine: Mix the dry and wet ingredients together until just combined, ensuring all elements work harmoniously to avoid harm.
4. Cook: Heat a non-stick skillet and pour batter to form pancakes, cooking until bubbles form and then flipping, maintaining a safe and balanced approach.
5. Serve: Serve warm with healthy toppings like fresh fruit or a light drizzle of maple syrup, emphasizing the importance of preventing harm.

Recipe 4: Justice Parfait

Ingredients:

- 1 cup Greek yogurt (Fair access)
- 1/2 cup granola (Equitable resources)
- 1/2 cup mixed berries (Non-discrimination)
- 1 tablespoon chia seeds (Fair distribution)
- 1 teaspoon honey (Equality in care)

Instructions:

1. Layer Yogurt: Spoon a layer of Greek yogurt into a serving glass, representing fair access to healthcare.
2. Add Granola: Add a layer of granola, ensuring equitable resources are provided.

3. Top with Berries: Layer mixed berries, highlighting the importance of non-discrimination in treatment.
4. Sprinkle Chia Seeds: Sprinkle chia seeds on top, representing fair distribution of healthcare resources.
5. Drizzle Honey: Drizzle with honey for a touch of sweetness, emphasizing equality in care.
6. Serve: Serve immediately, illustrating the principle of justice in a balanced and fair presentation.

Recipe 5: Confidentiality Cereal Bowl

Ingredients:

- 1 cup whole grain cereal (Protecting information)
- 1/2 cup sliced bananas (Privacy)
- 1/2 cup sliced strawberries (Trust)
- 1 tablespoon flax seeds (Security)

- 1 cup low-fat milk (Respecting confidentiality)

Instructions:

1. Prepare Cereal: Pour whole grain cereal into a bowl, symbolizing the foundation of protecting patient information.
2. Add Bananas: Top with sliced bananas, representing the privacy of patient details.
3. Include Strawberries: Add sliced strawberries, fostering trust between patient and provider.
4. Sprinkle Flax Seeds: Sprinkle flax seeds on top, ensuring security and protection of sensitive information.
5. Pour Milk: Pour low-fat milk over the cereal, respecting confidentiality in all aspects of care.

6. Serve: Serve immediately, maintaining the integrity and confidentiality of patient information in every bite.

Recipe 6: Integrity Frittata

Ingredients:

- 6 large eggs (Honesty)
- 1/4 cup milk (Transparency)
- 1/2 cup diced tomatoes (Truthfulness)
- 1/2 cup chopped spinach (Accountability)
- 1/4 cup feta cheese (Ethical standards)
- Salt and pepper to taste (Professionalism)

Instructions:

1. Whisk Eggs: Crack the eggs into a bowl, add milk, and whisk together, representing honesty and transparency in healthcare.
2. Prepare Vegetables: Dice tomatoes and chop spinach, ensuring all ingredients are fresh and truthful.
3. Combine: Mix the tomatoes and spinach into the eggs, adding feta cheese, embodying accountability and adherence to ethical standards.
4. Season: Add salt and pepper to taste, maintaining a professional approach.
5. Cook: Pour the mixture into a heated, non-stick skillet and cook on medium heat until the edges are set. Then transfer to a preheated oven and bake until the frittata is fully cooked.
6. Serve: Slice and serve warm, highlighting the integrity in every step of patient care.

Recipe 7: Compassionate Breakfast Burrito

Ingredients:

- 1 whole wheat tortilla (Empathy)
- 2 large eggs (Understanding)
- 1/4 cup black beans (Support)
- 1/4 cup diced bell peppers (Sensitivity)
- 1/4 cup shredded cheese (Care)
- Salsa (Communication)

Instructions:

1. Scramble Eggs: Whisk the eggs and cook them in a non-stick skillet, representing understanding in patient care.
2. Prepare Filling: Warm the black beans and dice the bell peppers, ensuring support and sensitivity to patient needs.

3. Combine Ingredients: Place the scrambled eggs, black beans, and bell peppers in the center of the tortilla, adding shredded cheese to symbolize care.
4. Wrap: Fold the sides of the tortilla over the filling and roll it up tightly.
5. Serve with Salsa: Serve with a side of salsa to promote open communication and connection with patients.

Recipe 8: Dignity French Toast

Ingredients:

- 2 slices of whole grain bread (Respect)
- 2 large eggs (Humanity)
- 1/4 cup milk (Kindness)
- 1 teaspoon vanilla extract (Dignity)
- 1 teaspoon cinnamon (Empowerment)
- Fresh berries (Upholding honor)

Instructions:

1. Prepare Mixture: Whisk together eggs, milk, vanilla extract, and cinnamon in a bowl, representing a blend of humanity, kindness, and dignity.
2. Dip Bread: Dip each slice of bread into the mixture, ensuring it is fully coated, symbolizing respect and empowerment.
3. Cook: Heat a non-stick skillet and cook the bread slices until golden brown on both sides.
4. Serve: Top with fresh berries and serve, emphasizing the importance of upholding the honor and dignity of patients in every aspect of care.

Recipe 9: Confidentiality Yogurt Bowl

Ingredients:

- 1 cup plain Greek yogurt (Protecting patient information)
- 1/2 cup granola (Trust)
- 1/4 cup blueberries (Discretion)
- 1 tablespoon honey (Security)
- 1 tablespoon chia seeds (Confidentiality)

Instructions:

1. Prepare Base: Spoon Greek yogurt into a bowl, representing the foundation of protecting patient information.
2. Add Granola: Sprinkle granola on top, symbolizing the trust built with patients.
3. Top with Blueberries: Add blueberries for discretion and careful handling of sensitive information.

4. Drizzle Honey: Drizzle honey over the bowl, ensuring the security of patient details.
5. Sprinkle Chia Seeds: Finish with chia seeds, upholding the principle of confidentiality in patient care.

Recipe 10: Advocacy Avocado Toast

Ingredients:

- 1 ripe avocado (Supporting patient rights)
- 2 slices whole grain bread (Empowerment)
- 1 tablespoon lemon juice (Championing needs)
- Salt and pepper to taste (Encouragement)
- 1/4 cup cherry tomatoes (Patient voice)
- Red pepper flakes (Strength)

Instructions:

1. Toast Bread: Toast the whole grain bread slices, representing the empowerment of patients.
2. Prepare Avocado: Mash the avocado in a bowl, mixing in lemon juice, salt, and pepper to symbolize supporting and championing patient rights and needs.
3. Spread: Spread the mashed avocado evenly on the toasted bread, ensuring each patient's voice is heard and respected.
4. Top with Tomatoes: Add halved cherry tomatoes on top, highlighting the importance of including the patient's perspective.
5. Season: Sprinkle with red pepper flakes for added strength and encouragement.

6. Serve: Serve immediately, advocating for the patient's best interests in a nourishing and supportive manner.

Chapter 5: LUNCH RECIPES

Recipe 1: Informed Consent Salad

Ingredients:

- 2 cups mixed greens (Transparency)
- 1/2 cup cherry tomatoes (Understanding)
- 1/4 cup sliced cucumbers (Patient education)
- 1/4 cup shredded carrots (Clarity)
- 1/4 cup feta cheese (Voluntariness)
- 1/4 cup sunflower seeds (Comprehensive information)
- Olive oil and balsamic vinegar (Communication)

Instructions:

1. Prepare Greens: Place the mixed greens in a large salad bowl, representing the foundation of transparency in the patient-provider relationship.
2. Add Vegetables: Add cherry tomatoes, sliced cucumbers, and shredded carrots, symbolizing the understanding and clarity necessary for informed consent.
3. Include Cheese and Seeds: Sprinkle feta cheese and sunflower seeds over the salad, embodying the principles of voluntariness and providing comprehensive information.
4. Mix Dressing: Combine olive oil and balsamic vinegar in a small bowl, emphasizing clear and effective communication.
5. Toss Salad: Drizzle the dressing over the salad and toss well, ensuring that

all components work together to support informed consent.
6. Serve: Serve immediately, highlighting the importance of ensuring patients are fully informed and voluntary in their healthcare decisions.

Recipe 2: Beneficence Buddha Bowl

Ingredients:

- 1 cup cooked quinoa (Promoting well-being)
- 1/2 cup steamed broccoli (Health benefits)
- 1/2 cup roasted sweet potatoes (Positive outcomes)
- 1/4 cup chickpeas (Support)
- 1/4 avocado, sliced (Holistic care)
- 2 tablespoons tahini dressing (Compassion)

- 1 tablespoon chopped parsley (Enhancement)

Instructions:

1. Prepare Base: Place the cooked quinoa in the bottom of a bowl, symbolizing the foundation of promoting well-being in patient care.
2. Add Vegetables: Add steamed broccoli and roasted sweet potatoes to the bowl, focusing on treatments and interventions that provide health benefits and positive outcomes.
3. Include Chickpeas and Avocado: Add chickpeas and sliced avocado, representing holistic care and support for the patient.
4. Drizzle Dressing: Drizzle tahini dressing over the bowl, embodying compassion in the care provided.

5. Garnish: Sprinkle chopped parsley on top to enhance the presentation and benefits.
6. Serve: Serve immediately, showcasing the commitment to the patient's well-being in every aspect of their care.

Recipe 3: Non-maleficence Veggie Wrap

Ingredients:

- 1 whole wheat wrap (Avoiding harm)
- 1/4 cup hummus (Preventing risks)
- 1/2 cup spinach (Safety)
- 1/4 cup shredded carrots (Minimizing risks)
- 1/4 cup sliced bell peppers (Patient safety)
- 1/4 cup sliced cucumbers (Careful consideration)

- Salt and pepper to taste (Prudent judgment)

Instructions:

1. Spread Hummus: Spread a layer of hummus over the whole wheat wrap, representing the commitment to avoiding harm.
2. Add Spinach: Place spinach leaves evenly over the hummus, focusing on patient safety.
3. Include Vegetables: Add shredded carrots, sliced bell peppers, and sliced cucumbers, ensuring all actions minimize risks to the patient.
4. Season: Sprinkle with salt and pepper to taste, using prudent judgment in every step.
5. Wrap: Roll up the wrap tightly, ensuring all components are secure and safe.

6. Serve: Slice in half and serve, emphasizing the importance of non-maleficence in patient care.

Recipe 4: Justice Grain Bowl

Ingredients:

- 1 cup brown rice (Fair access)
- 1/2 cup black beans (Equity)
- 1/2 cup corn kernels (Equality)
- 1/4 cup diced red onion (Fair treatment)
- 1/4 cup diced bell peppers (Non-discrimination)
- 1/4 cup salsa (Inclusivity)
- 1/4 cup shredded lettuce (Balance)
- 2 tablespoons lime juice (Fair distribution)

Instructions:

1. Prepare Base: Place the cooked brown rice in a bowl, representing fair access to healthcare resources.
2. Add Beans and Corn: Add black beans and corn kernels, ensuring equity and equality in the care provided.
3. Include Vegetables: Add diced red onion and bell peppers, symbolizing fair treatment and non-discrimination.
4. Top with Salsa: Spoon salsa over the bowl, promoting inclusivity and respect for all patients.
5. Garnish: Add shredded lettuce and drizzle lime juice over the top, maintaining balance and fair distribution in healthcare.
6. Serve: Serve immediately, showcasing justice in every aspect of patient care.

Recipe 5: Confidentiality Chicken Salad

Ingredients:

- 1 cup shredded cooked chicken (Protecting patient information)
- 1/4 cup diced celery (Privacy)
- 1/4 cup diced apples (Trust)
- 1/4 cup dried cranberries (Discretion)
- 2 tablespoons mayonnaise (Security)
- 1 tablespoon lemon juice (Confidential handling)
- Salt and pepper to taste (Respect for privacy)
- Whole wheat bread or lettuce leaves for serving (Choices in confidentiality)

Instructions:

1. Prepare Chicken: Place the shredded chicken in a bowl, symbolizing the protection of patient information.
2. Add Vegetables and Fruit: Add diced celery, apples, and dried cranberries, ensuring privacy and trust in the patient-provider relationship.

3. Mix Dressing: In a separate bowl, combine mayonnaise and lemon juice, representing secure and confidential handling of information.
4. Combine: Mix the dressing with the chicken and vegetable mixture, ensuring all elements are handled with care and respect for privacy.
5. Season: Add salt and pepper to taste, maintaining respect for the confidentiality of patient information.
6. Serve: Serve the chicken salad on whole wheat bread or lettuce leaves, offering choices that respect confidentiality.

Recipe 6: Respect Stir-Fry

Ingredients:

- 1 cup cooked brown rice (Respect for cultural diversity)

- 1/2 cup sliced bell peppers (Listening)
- 1/2 cup snap peas (Understanding)
- 1/2 cup broccoli florets (Acknowledgment)
- 1/4 cup sliced carrots (Sensitivity)
- 1/4 cup sliced onions (Empathy)
- 2 tablespoons soy sauce (Honoring preferences)
- 1 tablespoon olive oil (Thoughtfulness)
- Sesame seeds for garnish (Recognizing individuality)

Instructions:

1. Prepare Vegetables: Slice bell peppers, snap peas, broccoli, carrots, and onions, representing the need to listen, understand, and acknowledge patients' diverse backgrounds and preferences.

2. Heat Oil: Heat olive oil in a large pan over medium heat, symbolizing thoughtfulness in patient care.
3. Stir-Fry Vegetables: Add the vegetables to the pan and stir-fry for 5-7 minutes until tender, ensuring sensitivity and empathy throughout the process.
4. Add Sauce: Pour in the soy sauce and mix well, honoring patients' preferences and cultural diversity.
5. Combine with Rice: Add the cooked brown rice and stir to combine everything evenly.
6. Garnish and Serve: Sprinkle sesame seeds on top and serve immediately, recognizing and respecting each patient's individuality.

Recipe 7: Compassion Lentil Soup

Ingredients:

- 1 cup dried lentils (Compassion)
- 1 chopped onion (Empathy)
- 2 minced garlic cloves (Care)
- 1 diced carrot (Kindness)
- 1 diced celery stalk (Understanding)
- 4 cups vegetable broth (Support)
- 1 teaspoon cumin (Warmth)
- 1 teaspoon paprika (Comfort)
- Salt and pepper to taste (Sympathy)
- 1 tablespoon olive oil (Nurturing)
- Fresh parsley for garnish (Encouragement)

Instructions:

1. Prepare Ingredients: Chop the onion, carrot, and celery, and mince the garlic, symbolizing empathy, care, and understanding.
2. Heat Oil: In a large pot, heat olive oil over medium heat, representing nurturing and support.

3. Sauté Vegetables: Add the onion, garlic, carrot, and celery to the pot, sautéing until softened, embodying compassion and kindness.
4. Add Lentils and Broth: Stir in the lentils and pour in the vegetable broth, ensuring the mixture provides warmth and comfort.
5. Season: Add cumin, paprika, salt, and pepper, maintaining sympathy and thoughtful seasoning.
6. Cook: Bring to a boil, then reduce heat and let simmer for 30-35 minutes until lentils are tender.
7. Serve: Ladle into bowls, garnish with fresh parsley, and serve, offering encouragement and continuous care.

Recipe 8: Integrity Quinoa Salad

Ingredients:

- 1 cup cooked quinoa (Honesty)
- 1/2 cup chickpeas (Accountability)
- 1/2 cup diced cucumber (Transparency)
- 1/4 cup diced red onion (Truthfulness)
- 1/4 cup crumbled feta cheese (Ethical standards)
- 1/4 cup chopped fresh mint (Moral integrity)
- 2 tablespoons olive oil (Trust)
- 1 tablespoon lemon juice (Openness)
- Salt and pepper to taste (Responsibility)

Instructions:

1. Prepare Quinoa: Cook quinoa according to package instructions and let it cool, symbolizing the foundation of honesty in healthcare.
2. Combine Ingredients: In a large bowl, combine quinoa, chickpeas, cucumber,

red onion, and feta cheese, ensuring all components reflect accountability, transparency, and truthfulness.
3. Add Fresh Mint: Chop and add fresh mint, representing moral integrity.
4. Mix Dressing: In a small bowl, whisk together olive oil and lemon juice, emphasizing trust and openness.
5. Season: Add salt and pepper to taste, maintaining responsibility in every step.
6. Toss and Serve: Toss the salad with the dressing and serve immediately, showcasing integrity in patient care and decision-making.

Recipe 9: Advocacy Veggie Sandwich

Ingredients:

- 2 slices whole grain bread (Advocacy)
- 1/4 cup hummus (Support)

- 1/4 cup sliced avocado (Championing patient needs)
- 1/4 cup shredded lettuce (Representation)
- 1/4 cup sliced tomatoes (Listening)
- 1/4 cup sliced cucumbers (Empowering)
- Salt and pepper to taste (Strength)
- Olive oil (Encouragement)

Instructions:

1. Toast Bread: Lightly toast the whole grain bread slices, representing advocacy for patient rights and needs.
2. Spread Hummus: Evenly spread hummus on one side of each slice of bread, providing a foundation of support.
3. Layer Vegetables: Layer avocado, shredded lettuce, sliced tomatoes, and sliced cucumbers on one slice of

bread, symbolizing listening, empowering, and representing the patient.
4. Season: Sprinkle with salt and pepper to taste, adding strength and encouragement.
5. Assemble Sandwich: Top with the other slice of bread, hummus side down.
6. Serve: Cut in half and serve, championing patient needs and advocacy through thoughtful, supportive care.

Recipe 10: Trust Tacos

Ingredients:

- 4 small whole wheat tortillas (Building trust)
- 1 cup cooked black beans (Reliability)
- 1/2 cup corn kernels (Honesty)

- 1/4 cup diced red onion (Transparency)
- 1/4 cup chopped cilantro (Consistency)
- 1/4 cup crumbled queso fresco (Dependability)
- Lime wedges (Clarity)
- Salt and pepper to taste (Trustworthiness)
- Hot sauce (Openness)

Instructions:

1. Prepare Tortillas: Warm the whole wheat tortillas in a dry skillet, symbolizing the foundation of building trust.
2. Prepare Filling: In a bowl, mix cooked black beans, corn kernels, and diced red onion, representing reliability, honesty, and transparency.

3. Season: Add salt and pepper to taste, ensuring trustworthiness in the mix.
4. Assemble Tacos: Divide the bean mixture evenly among the tortillas.
5. Garnish: Top with chopped cilantro and crumbled queso fresco, representing consistency and dependability.
6. Serve: Serve with lime wedges and a drizzle of hot sauce for added clarity and openness, reinforcing the importance of trust in patient care.

Chapter 6: DINNER RECIPES

Recipe 1: Autonomy Stir-Fry

Ingredients:

- 1 cup tofu or chicken, cubed (Patient's choice)

- 2 cups mixed vegetables (bell peppers, broccoli, snap peas) (Patient's preferences)
- 2 tablespoons soy sauce (Informed consent)
- 1 tablespoon sesame oil (Supportive environment)
- 1 tablespoon minced garlic (Clear communication)
- 1 tablespoon minced ginger (Understanding)
- 1 cup cooked rice (Foundation of care)
- Sesame seeds for garnish (Respect)

Instructions:

1. Prepare Protein: Choose tofu or chicken based on patient preferences, symbolizing respect for patient autonomy.

2. Heat Oil: In a large pan, heat sesame oil over medium heat, creating a supportive environment.
3. Sauté Garlic and Ginger: Add minced garlic and ginger, representing clear communication and understanding.
4. Cook Protein: Add the cubed tofu or chicken and cook until browned, ensuring the patient's choices are honored.
5. Add Vegetables: Add the mixed vegetables to the pan, incorporating the patient's preferences.
6. Season: Pour in soy sauce and stir well, representing informed consent.
7. Combine: Serve the stir-fry over a bed of cooked rice, establishing a foundation of care.
8. Garnish: Sprinkle with sesame seeds and serve immediately, emphasizing respect for patient autonomy in every aspect.

Recipe 2: Beneficence Baked Salmon

Ingredients:

- 4 salmon fillets (Promoting well-being)
- 2 tablespoons olive oil (Caring)
- 1 tablespoon lemon juice (Enhancing quality of life)
- 2 cloves garlic, minced (Preventing harm)
- 1 teaspoon dried dill (Encouraging health)
- Salt and pepper to taste (Ensuring safety)
- Steamed asparagus (Supportive care)
- Quinoa or brown rice (Nourishment)

Instructions:

1. Preheat Oven: Preheat your oven to 375°F (190°C), creating a safe and caring environment for cooking.
2. Prepare Marinade: In a small bowl, mix olive oil, lemon juice, minced garlic, dill, salt, and pepper, focusing on ingredients that enhance well-being.
3. Marinate Salmon: Place salmon fillets on a baking sheet and brush with the marinade, ensuring the fish is well-coated.
4. Bake Salmon: Bake in the preheated oven for 15-20 minutes, or until the salmon is cooked through and flakes easily with a fork.
5. Prepare Sides: While the salmon is baking, steam asparagus and cook quinoa or brown rice to serve alongside, promoting a holistic approach to health.
6. Serve: Plate the salmon with asparagus and quinoa or brown rice, highlighting the importance of

beneficence in providing nutritious and health-promoting meals.

Recipe 3: Non-maleficence Veggie Pasta

Ingredients:

- 12 ounces whole wheat pasta (Avoiding harm)
- 2 cups cherry tomatoes, halved (Healthful choices)
- 1 cup spinach (Safety)
- 1/4 cup olive oil (Careful consideration)
- 3 cloves garlic, minced (Preventing risks)
- 1/2 teaspoon red pepper flakes (Balanced intervention)
- 1/4 cup grated Parmesan cheese (Positive outcomes)
- Salt and pepper to taste (Prudent judgment)

Instructions:

1. Cook Pasta: Cook the whole wheat pasta according to package instructions, representing the commitment to making healthful choices.
2. Prepare Vegetables: In a large skillet, heat olive oil over medium heat and sauté minced garlic until fragrant, ensuring safety and preventing risks.
3. Add Tomatoes and Spinach: Add cherry tomatoes and spinach, cooking until the tomatoes are soft and the spinach is wilted, embodying balanced intervention.
4. Combine: Drain the pasta and add it to the skillet, tossing to combine all ingredients.
5. Season: Sprinkle with red pepper flakes, salt, and pepper, using prudent judgment to season.

6. Serve: Plate the pasta and top with grated Parmesan cheese, emphasizing non-maleficence by providing a delicious, balanced, and safe meal.

Recipe 4: Justice Stuffed Peppers

Ingredients:

- 4 large bell peppers (Fair access)
- 1 cup cooked quinoa (Equity)
- 1 cup black beans (Equality)
- 1/2 cup corn kernels (Non-discrimination)
- 1/2 cup diced tomatoes (Inclusivity)
- 1/4 cup diced red onion (Fair treatment)
- 1 teaspoon cumin (Balance)
- 1/2 teaspoon paprika (Respect)
- 1/4 cup shredded cheese (Support)
- Salt and pepper to taste (Justice)

Instructions:

1. Preheat Oven: Preheat your oven to 375°F (190°C), creating an environment that promotes fairness and balance.
2. Prepare Peppers: Cut the tops off the bell peppers and remove the seeds, symbolizing fair access.
3. Mix Filling: In a bowl, combine cooked quinoa, black beans, corn, diced tomatoes, red onion, cumin, paprika, salt, and pepper, ensuring equity, equality, and non-discrimination.
4. Stuff Peppers: Fill each bell pepper with the quinoa mixture, packing it well.
5. Bake Peppers: Place the stuffed peppers in a baking dish and cover with foil. Bake for 30 minutes, then remove the foil, sprinkle with cheese, and bake for another 10 minutes.

6. Serve: Plate the stuffed peppers and serve, emphasizing justice in ensuring all patients receive fair and inclusive care.

Recipe 5: Confidentiality Chicken Enchiladas

Ingredients:

- 2 cups shredded cooked chicken (Protecting patient information)
- 1 cup enchilada sauce (Privacy)
- 8 small whole wheat tortillas (Trust)
- 1/2 cup diced onions (Discretion)
- 1 cup shredded cheese (Security)
- 1/4 cup chopped cilantro (Confidential handling)
- 1/4 cup sour cream (Respect for confidentiality)
- Salt and pepper to taste (Responsibility)

Instructions:

1. Preheat Oven: Preheat your oven to 350°F (175°C), ensuring a secure and controlled environment.
2. Prepare Filling: In a bowl, mix shredded chicken, half of the enchilada sauce, diced onions, salt, and pepper, symbolizing the careful handling of patient information.
3. Fill Tortillas: Spoon the chicken mixture onto each tortilla and roll up, maintaining discretion and privacy.
4. Assemble Enchiladas: Place the rolled tortillas seam-side down in a baking dish, ensuring they are secure and protected.
5. Add Sauce and Cheese: Pour the remaining enchilada sauce over the top and sprinkle with shredded cheese, symbolizing security and respect for confidentiality.

6. Bake: Cover the dish with foil and bake for 20 minutes, then remove the foil and bake for an additional 10 minutes until the cheese is melted and bubbly.
7. Serve: Garnish with chopped cilantro and a dollop of sour cream, and serve, emphasizing the importance of confidentiality and trust in patient care.

Recipe 6: Fidelity Meatloaf

Ingredients:

- 1 pound ground beef or turkey (Commitment)
- 1/2 cup breadcrumbs (Dependability)
- 1/4 cup finely chopped onion (Honesty)
- 1/4 cup finely chopped green bell pepper (Loyalty)

- 1/4 cup ketchup (Consistency)
- 1 egg (Trust)
- 2 cloves garlic, minced (Support)
- 1 teaspoon Worcestershire sauce (Integrity)
- Salt and pepper to taste (Faithfulness)
- 1/4 cup ketchup for topping (Ongoing support)

Instructions:

1. Preheat Oven: Preheat your oven to 375°F (190°C), creating a consistent environment.
2. Mix Ingredients: In a large bowl, combine the ground meat, breadcrumbs, onion, green bell pepper, ketchup, egg, minced garlic, Worcestershire sauce, salt, and pepper. Mix well, ensuring all components are integrated,

symbolizing the integration of honesty, loyalty, and integrity.
3. Form Meatloaf: Shape the mixture into a loaf and place it in a baking dish, representing the firm commitment to the principles.
4. Top with Ketchup: Spread 1/4 cup of ketchup on top, symbolizing ongoing support.
5. Bake: Bake in the preheated oven for 50-60 minutes, or until fully cooked, ensuring dependability and consistency.
6. Serve: Let the meatloaf rest for a few minutes before slicing and serving, emphasizing trust and faithfulness in the caregiving relationship.

Recipe 7: Non-maleficence Mushroom Risotto

Ingredients:

- 1 cup Arborio rice (Safe practices)
- 4 cups vegetable broth (Protecting patients)
- 1 cup sliced mushrooms (Minimizing harm)
- 1/2 cup finely chopped onion (Careful attention)
- 2 cloves garlic, minced (Preventing risks)
- 1/2 cup grated Parmesan cheese (Positive outcomes)
- 1/4 cup white wine (Moderation)
- 2 tablespoons olive oil (Caution)
- Salt and pepper to taste (Prudent judgment)
- Fresh parsley for garnish (Ethical considerations)

Instructions:

1. Heat Broth: In a saucepan, bring the vegetable broth to a simmer and keep

it warm, symbolizing ongoing protection.
2. Sauté Vegetables: In a large pan, heat olive oil over medium heat. Add the onion and garlic, cooking until softened, emphasizing careful attention and preventing risks.
3. Cook Mushrooms: Add the sliced mushrooms and cook until tender, representing the minimization of harm.
4. Toast Rice: Add the Arborio rice to the pan and cook for 1-2 minutes, ensuring it is well-coated with oil, symbolizing safe practices.
5. Add Wine: Pour in the white wine and cook until absorbed, practicing moderation.
6. Add Broth Gradually: Add the warm broth one ladle at a time, stirring constantly and allowing each addition to be absorbed before adding more. Continue until the rice is creamy and cooked through.

7. Finish with Cheese: Stir in the Parmesan cheese, adding salt and pepper to taste, and ensuring a positive outcome.
8. Serve: Garnish with fresh parsley and serve immediately, focusing on ethical considerations and non-maleficence.

Recipe 8: Veracity Vegetable Lasagna

Ingredients:

- 9 lasagna noodles (Truthfulness)
- 2 cups ricotta cheese (Transparency)
- 2 cups shredded mozzarella cheese (Honesty)
- 1/2 cup grated Parmesan cheese (Clarity)
- 1 egg (Sincerity)
- 1 jar marinara sauce (Consistency)
- 1 cup chopped spinach (Straightforwardness)

- 1 cup sliced mushrooms (Trustworthiness)
- 1/2 cup chopped zucchini (Clear communication)
- 2 cloves garlic, minced (Integrity)
- Salt and pepper to taste (Accuracy)
- Fresh basil for garnish (Upholding truth)

Instructions:

1. Preheat Oven: Preheat your oven to 375°F (190°C), creating a clear and consistent environment.
2. Cook Noodles: Cook the lasagna noodles according to package instructions, drain, and set aside, symbolizing the foundation of truthfulness.
3. Prepare Filling: In a bowl, mix ricotta cheese, egg, salt, and pepper until

smooth, representing transparency and honesty.
4. Sauté Vegetables: In a large pan, heat a little oil over medium heat. Add minced garlic, spinach, mushrooms, and zucchini, cooking until tender, ensuring straightforwardness and clear communication.
5. Assemble Lasagna: Spread a thin layer of marinara sauce on the bottom of a baking dish. Layer 3 lasagna noodles over the sauce, followed by half of the ricotta mixture, half of the sautéed vegetables, and a third of the mozzarella cheese. Repeat the layers, ending with the remaining noodles and sauce, and top with the remaining mozzarella and Parmesan cheese.
6. Bake: Cover with foil and bake for 30 minutes. Remove the foil and bake for an additional 10-15 minutes, until the cheese is bubbly and golden.
7. Serve: Garnish with fresh basil and serve, emphasizing veracity by

upholding truth and integrity in the meal.

Recipe 9: Dignity Roast Chicken

Ingredients:

- 1 whole chicken (Respect)
- 1 tablespoon olive oil (Care)
- 2 cloves garlic, minced (Compassion)
- 1 lemon, halved (Empathy)
- Fresh rosemary sprigs (Honor)
- Salt and pepper to taste (Self-worth)
- Mixed roasted vegetables (Supporting dignity)

Instructions:

1. Preheat Oven: Preheat your oven to 375°F (190°C), ensuring a respectful environment.
2. Prepare Chicken: Rub the chicken with olive oil, minced garlic, salt, and pepper, ensuring it is well-coated with care and compassion.
3. Stuff Chicken: Place the halved lemon and rosemary sprigs inside the cavity of the chicken, symbolizing empathy and honor.
4. Roast Chicken: Place the chicken in a roasting pan and roast in the preheated oven for 1.5-2 hours, or until the internal temperature reaches 165°F (74°C). Baste occasionally with the pan juices.
5. Prepare Vegetables: Toss mixed vegetables with olive oil, salt, and pepper, and spread them around the chicken in the roasting pan, supporting dignity through thoughtful preparation.

6. Serve: Let the chicken rest for a few minutes before carving and serving with the roasted vegetables, emphasizing the respect and self-worth given to the patient through dignified care.

Recipe 10: Accountability Stuffed Eggplant

Ingredients:

- 2 large eggplants (Responsibility)
- 1 cup cooked quinoa (Reliability)
- 1/2 cup diced tomatoes (Transparency)
- 1/2 cup chickpeas (Honesty)
- 1/4 cup diced onions (Answerability)
- 2 cloves garlic, minced (Ethical responsibility)
- 1/4 cup chopped parsley (Commitment)

- 1/4 cup shredded cheese (Accountable actions)
- Salt and pepper to taste (Dependability)
- Olive oil (Support)

Instructions:

1. Preheat Oven: Preheat your oven to 375°F (190°C), establishing a reliable environment.
2. Prepare Eggplants: Cut the eggplants in half lengthwise and scoop out the flesh, leaving a 1/2-inch border. Chop the scooped-out flesh and set aside, symbolizing the core of responsibility.
3. Sauté Filling: In a pan, heat olive oil over medium heat. Add diced onions, minced garlic, and the chopped eggplant flesh, cooking until tender. Add diced tomatoes and chickpeas, cooking for a few more minutes.

4. Combine Ingredients: In a bowl, combine the cooked quinoa, sautéed vegetables, salt, pepper, and chopped parsley, ensuring all components represent reliability, honesty, and answerability.
5. Stuff Eggplants: Fill each eggplant half with the quinoa mixture, packing it well.
6. Bake: Place the stuffed eggplants on a baking sheet and top with shredded cheese. Bake in the preheated oven for 25-30 minutes, or until the eggplants are tender and the cheese is melted.
7. Serve: Serve immediately, emphasizing accountability through the thoughtful and ethical preparation of the meal.

Chapter 7: SNACKS RECIPES

Recipe 1: Autonomy Energy Bites

Ingredients:

- 1 cup rolled oats (Empowerment)
- 1/2 cup peanut butter (Respect for choices)
- 1/3 cup honey (Trust)
- 1/2 cup mini chocolate chips (Freedom)
- 1/2 cup flaxseeds (Informed decision-making)
- 1 teaspoon vanilla extract (Support)
- Pinch of salt (Balance)

Instructions:

1. Combine Ingredients: In a large bowl, mix together the rolled oats, peanut butter, honey, mini chocolate chips, flaxseeds, vanilla extract, and a pinch of salt, ensuring all ingredients are well incorporated to symbolize empowerment and respect for choices.
2. Chill Mixture: Place the mixture in the refrigerator for about 30 minutes to

make it easier to handle, representing the supportive environment needed for informed decision-making.
3. Form Bites: Once chilled, roll the mixture into small, bite-sized balls, emphasizing balance and trust.
4. Store and Serve: Store the energy bites in an airtight container in the refrigerator. Enjoy them as a snack, highlighting the principle of autonomy by allowing individuals to make their own choices about when and how to enjoy their snacks.

Recipe 2: Beneficence Fruit and Nut Mix

Ingredients:

- 1 cup almonds (Nourishment)
- 1 cup cashews (Well-being)
- 1/2 cup dried cranberries (Health promotion)

- 1/2 cup dried apricots (Care)
- 1/4 cup pumpkin seeds (Protection)
- 1/4 cup dark chocolate chips (Positive outcomes)

Instructions:

1. Combine Ingredients: In a large bowl, combine the almonds, cashews, dried cranberries, dried apricots, pumpkin seeds, and dark chocolate chips, ensuring all components are mixed well to symbolize nourishment and well-being.
2. Store Mix: Store the mix in an airtight container, representing continuous care and protection.
3. Serve: Serve the fruit and nut mix as a snack, emphasizing beneficence by promoting health and well-being through a nutritious and delicious option.

Recipe 3: Non-maleficence Veggie Sticks with Hummus

Ingredients:

- 1 cup baby carrots (Prevention of harm)
- 1 cup cucumber sticks (Safety)
- 1 cup bell pepper strips (Minimizing risks)
- 1 cup celery sticks (Careful consideration)
- 1 cup hummus (Healthy choice)

Instructions:

1. Prepare Vegetables: Wash and cut the baby carrots, cucumbers, bell peppers, and celery into sticks, ensuring they

are ready to eat, symbolizing the prevention of harm and safety.
2. Serve with Hummus: Arrange the vegetable sticks on a platter with a bowl of hummus in the center, representing minimizing risks and careful consideration.
3. Enjoy: Serve as a healthy snack, highlighting non-maleficence by providing a nutritious, safe, and risk-free option.

Recipe 4: Justice Apple Slices with Almond Butter

Ingredients:

- 2 apples, sliced (Equity)
- 1/2 cup almond butter (Fairness)
- 1 tablespoon honey (Inclusivity)
- 1 tablespoon chia seeds (Balance)

Instructions:

1. Slice Apples: Wash and slice the apples into wedges, ensuring even and fair portions, symbolizing equity.
2. Prepare Almond Butter: In a small bowl, mix the almond butter with honey until well combined, representing fairness and inclusivity.
3. Serve with Seeds: Arrange the apple slices on a plate and sprinkle chia seeds over the almond butter for added nutrition and balance.
4. Enjoy: Serve as a snack, highlighting justice by ensuring everyone has access to a nutritious and fair snack option.

Recipe 5: Confidentiality Greek Yogurt Parfait

Ingredients:

- 1 cup Greek yogurt (Privacy)
- 1/2 cup granola (Trust)
- 1/2 cup mixed berries (Respect)
- 1 tablespoon honey (Security)
- 1 teaspoon chia seeds (Confidentiality)

Instructions:

1. Layer Ingredients: In a clear glass or bowl, layer half of the Greek yogurt, followed by half of the granola, and then half of the mixed berries. Repeat the layers, symbolizing the careful and respectful handling of confidential information.
2. Drizzle Honey: Drizzle honey over the top layer, representing the sweet aspect of maintaining trust and security.
3. Sprinkle Seeds: Sprinkle chia seeds on top, emphasizing confidentiality.

4. Serve: Serve immediately or refrigerate for later, highlighting the importance of maintaining privacy and respect in all interactions.

Recipe 6: Integrity Granola Bars

Ingredients:

- 2 cups rolled oats (Trustworthiness)
- 1 cup almond butter (Consistency)
- 1/2 cup honey (Transparency)
- 1/2 cup chopped nuts (Honesty)
- 1/2 cup dried fruit (Dependability)
- 1/4 cup dark chocolate chips (Commitment)
- 1 teaspoon vanilla extract (Sincerity)
- 1/4 teaspoon salt (Fairness)

Instructions:

1. Combine Ingredients: In a large bowl, mix together the rolled oats, almond butter, honey, chopped nuts, dried fruit, dark chocolate chips, vanilla extract, and salt until well combined, symbolizing trustworthiness and consistency.
2. Press into Pan: Line a baking dish with parchment paper and press the mixture firmly into the dish, ensuring it is evenly distributed to represent transparency and fairness.
3. Chill: Refrigerate for at least 2 hours to allow the bars to set, emphasizing commitment and dependability.
4. Cut and Serve: Once set, cut into bars and serve, highlighting the principle of integrity by providing a consistent and reliable snack.

Recipe 7: Compassionate Caprese Skewers

Ingredients:

- 1 cup cherry tomatoes (Empathy)
- 1 cup mini mozzarella balls (Kindness)
- Fresh basil leaves (Caring)
- 2 tablespoons balsamic glaze (Support)
- Salt and pepper to taste (Understanding)
- Wooden skewers (Connection)

Instructions:

1. Assemble Skewers: On each wooden skewer, thread a cherry tomato, a basil leaf, and a mini mozzarella ball, repeating the pattern until the skewer is full, symbolizing empathy and kindness.
2. Season: Sprinkle with salt and pepper to taste, representing understanding.
3. Drizzle Glaze: Drizzle balsamic glaze over the skewers, adding a touch of support and care.

4. Serve: Arrange the skewers on a platter and serve immediately, emphasizing compassion through the thoughtful and caring preparation of the snack.

Recipe 8: Respectful Rice Cakes

Ingredients:

- 4 rice cakes (Recognition)
- 1/2 cup hummus (Consideration)
- 1/4 cup shredded carrots (Acknowledgment)
- 1/4 cup cucumber slices (Appreciation)
- 1/4 cup sliced avocado (Dignity)
- Salt and pepper to taste (Courtesy)

Instructions:

1. Prepare Toppings: Slice the cucumber and avocado, and shred the carrots, symbolizing recognition and consideration.
2. Spread Hummus: Spread a layer of hummus on each rice cake, representing acknowledgment.
3. Add Toppings: Top each rice cake with shredded carrots, cucumber slices, and avocado, emphasizing appreciation and dignity.
4. Season: Sprinkle with salt and pepper to taste, highlighting courtesy.
5. Serve: Serve immediately as a snack, demonstrating respect through the careful and considerate preparation.

Recipe 9: Justice Trail Mix

Ingredients:

- 1 cup almonds (Equality)

- 1 cup cashews (Fairness)
- 1/2 cup dried cherries (Inclusion)
- 1/2 cup dried blueberries (Non-discrimination)
- 1/4 cup sunflower seeds (Balance)
- 1/4 cup dark chocolate chunks (Impartiality)

Instructions:

1. Combine Ingredients: In a large bowl, mix together the almonds, cashews, dried cherries, dried blueberries, sunflower seeds, and dark chocolate chunks, ensuring all components are well distributed to symbolize equality and fairness.
2. Mix Well: Stir the ingredients until they are evenly mixed, representing inclusion and non-discrimination.
3. Store and Serve: Store the trail mix in an airtight container and serve as a

snack, highlighting justice by ensuring everyone has access to a balanced and fair snack option.

Recipe 10: Confidentiality Yogurt Dip with Veggies

Ingredients:

- 1 cup Greek yogurt (Privacy)
- 1 tablespoon lemon juice (Discretion)
- 1 tablespoon chopped fresh dill (Trust)
- 1 teaspoon garlic powder (Security)
- Salt and pepper to taste (Confidential handling)
- Assorted fresh veggies (carrot sticks, cucumber slices, bell pepper strips) (Respect)

Instructions:

1. Prepare Dip: In a bowl, combine Greek yogurt, lemon juice, chopped dill, garlic powder, salt, and pepper, mixing well to symbolize privacy and discretion.
2. Serve with Veggies: Arrange the fresh veggies on a platter around the yogurt dip, representing respect and trust.
3. Enjoy: Serve immediately or refrigerate until ready to eat, emphasizing confidentiality by ensuring the dip is kept secure until served.

Chapter 8: DESSERT RECIPES

for medical Ethics in ingredients and instructions form

ChatGPT

Certainly! Here are five dessert recipes that metaphorically represent the principles of medical ethics:

Recipe 1: Autonomy Apple Crisp

Ingredients:

- 4 cups sliced apples (Empowerment)
- 1 tablespoon lemon juice (Informed choices)
- 1/2 cup granulated sugar (Trust)
- 1 teaspoon ground cinnamon (Respect)
- 1/2 cup rolled oats (Freedom)
- 1/2 cup flour (Support)
- 1/2 cup brown sugar (Responsibility)
- 1/4 cup melted butter (Guidance)

Instructions:

1. Preheat Oven: Preheat your oven to 350°F (175°C), creating a welcoming environment for decision-making.

2. Prepare Apples: In a bowl, toss the apple slices with lemon juice, granulated sugar, and cinnamon, ensuring the apples are evenly coated to symbolize empowerment and informed choices.
3. Make Topping: In another bowl, mix the oats, flour, brown sugar, and melted butter until crumbly, representing freedom and support.
4. Assemble Crisp: Spread the apples evenly in a baking dish and sprinkle the oat mixture on top, ensuring an even distribution of responsibility and guidance.
5. Bake: Bake for 30-35 minutes, or until the topping is golden brown and the apples are tender, emphasizing the balance of autonomy.
6. Serve: Let the apple crisp cool slightly before serving, highlighting the principle of autonomy by allowing individuals to choose when and how to enjoy their dessert.

Recipe 2: Beneficence Berry Parfait

Ingredients:

- 2 cups mixed berries (Health promotion)
- 2 cups Greek yogurt (Well-being)
- 1/2 cup granola (Nourishment)
- 2 tablespoons honey (Kindness)
- Fresh mint for garnish (Care)

Instructions:

1. Prepare Berries: Wash and prepare the mixed berries, ensuring they are fresh and ready to eat, symbolizing health promotion.
2. Layer Ingredients: In individual serving glasses, layer Greek yogurt, mixed berries, and granola, repeating the layers until the glasses are full,

representing well-being and nourishment.
3. Drizzle Honey: Drizzle honey over the top of each parfait, adding a touch of kindness.
4. Garnish: Garnish with fresh mint leaves, emphasizing care.
5. Serve: Serve immediately or refrigerate until ready to eat, highlighting beneficence by providing a delicious and healthy dessert option.

Recipe 3: Non-maleficence Chocolate Avocado Mousse

Ingredients:

- 2 ripe avocados (Minimizing harm)
- 1/4 cup cocoa powder (Preventing risks)
- 1/4 cup honey or maple syrup (Safe sweetness)

- 1 teaspoon vanilla extract (Careful consideration)
- Pinch of salt (Balance)
- Fresh berries for garnish (Positive outcomes)

Instructions:

1. Blend Ingredients: In a food processor, blend the avocados, cocoa powder, honey or maple syrup, vanilla extract, and salt until smooth and creamy, ensuring all ingredients are well incorporated to symbolize minimizing harm and preventing risks.
2. Chill Mousse: Transfer the mousse to serving bowls and refrigerate for at least 30 minutes to set, representing careful consideration and balance.

3. Garnish: Before serving, garnish with fresh berries, adding a touch of positive outcomes.
4. Serve: Serve chilled, highlighting non-maleficence by providing a safe and healthy dessert option.

Recipe 4: Justice Fruit Salad

Ingredients:

- 1 cup diced pineapple (Fairness)
- 1 cup diced mango (Equity)
- 1 cup sliced strawberries (Inclusivity)
- 1 cup blueberries (Non-discrimination)
- 1 kiwi, sliced (Impartiality)
- 1 tablespoon lime juice (Balance)
- 1 tablespoon honey (Integrity)

Instructions:

1. Prepare Fruit: Wash and prepare the fruit, ensuring even and fair portions, symbolizing fairness and equity.
2. Mix Fruit: In a large bowl, combine the pineapple, mango, strawberries, blueberries, and kiwi, mixing gently to ensure an even distribution of inclusivity and non-discrimination.
3. Add Dressing: In a small bowl, mix the lime juice and honey, then drizzle over the fruit salad, representing balance and integrity.
4. Toss and Serve: Toss the fruit salad gently to coat with the dressing and serve immediately, highlighting justice by ensuring everyone has access to a balanced and fair dessert.

Recipe 5: Fidelity Peanut Butter Cookies

Ingredients:

- 1 cup peanut butter (Commitment)
- 1/2 cup granulated sugar (Dependability)
- 1/2 cup brown sugar (Consistency)
- 1 egg (Trust)
- 1 teaspoon vanilla extract (Loyalty)
- 1/2 teaspoon baking soda (Support)
- Pinch of salt (Faithfulness)

Instructions:

1. Preheat Oven: Preheat your oven to 350°F (175°C), creating a consistent environment.
2. Mix Ingredients: In a large bowl, mix the peanut butter, granulated sugar, brown sugar, egg, vanilla extract, baking soda, and salt until well combined, symbolizing commitment, dependability, and consistency.
3. Form Cookies: Scoop tablespoons of dough onto a baking sheet lined with

parchment paper, flattening each with a fork to create a crisscross pattern, representing trust and loyalty.
4. Bake: Bake for 10-12 minutes, or until the edges are lightly golden, emphasizing support and faithfulness.
5. Cool and Serve: Let the cookies cool on the baking sheet for a few minutes before transferring to a wire rack to cool completely, highlighting fidelity by providing a dependable and consistent dessert.

Recipe 6: Respectful Raspberry Sorbet

Ingredients:

- 4 cups fresh raspberries (Acknowledgment)
- 1/2 cup sugar (Consideration)
- 1/2 cup water (Fairness)

- 1 tablespoon lemon juice (Recognition)
- Fresh mint for garnish (Appreciation)

Instructions:

1. Prepare Syrup: In a small saucepan, combine the sugar and water, heating until the sugar is dissolved to create a simple syrup, symbolizing consideration and fairness.
2. Blend Raspberries: In a blender, blend the raspberries and lemon juice until smooth, representing acknowledgment and recognition.
3. Combine Mixtures: Strain the raspberry puree to remove seeds, then mix the puree with the simple syrup, emphasizing appreciation.
4. Freeze: Pour the mixture into an ice cream maker and freeze according to the manufacturer's instructions.

Alternatively, pour into a shallow dish and freeze, stirring every 30 minutes until firm.

5. Serve: Scoop the sorbet into bowls and garnish with fresh mint, highlighting respect through the thoughtful and considerate preparation of the dessert.

Recipe 7: Integrity Chocolate Bark

Ingredients:

- 2 cups dark chocolate chips (Trustworthiness)
- 1/2 cup chopped almonds (Consistency)
- 1/4 cup dried cranberries (Transparency)
- 1/4 cup pumpkin seeds (Honesty)
- 1/4 cup shredded coconut (Sincerity)
- Pinch of sea salt (Fairness)

Instructions:

1. Melt Chocolate: In a microwave-safe bowl, melt the dark chocolate chips in 30-second intervals, stirring between each until smooth, representing trustworthiness and consistency.
2. Prepare Toppings: Mix the chopped almonds, dried cranberries, pumpkin seeds, and shredded coconut in a bowl, symbolizing transparency and honesty.
3. Spread Chocolate: Pour the melted chocolate onto a parchment-lined baking sheet, spreading it evenly with a spatula.
4. Add Toppings: Sprinkle the mixed toppings evenly over the melted chocolate and gently press them in. Add a pinch of sea salt for balance, representing fairness.
5. Set and Serve: Let the chocolate bark set in the refrigerator for about an

hour. Once set, break it into pieces and serve, emphasizing integrity through a consistent and reliable treat.

Recipe 8: Compassionate Carrot Cake Muffins

Ingredients:

- 1 cup grated carrots (Empathy)
- 1/2 cup applesauce (Kindness)
- 1/2 cup brown sugar (Care)
- 2 eggs (Support)
- 1 cup whole wheat flour (Understanding)
- 1 teaspoon baking powder (Patience)
- 1/2 teaspoon baking soda (Balance)
- 1 teaspoon ground cinnamon (Warmth)
- 1/2 teaspoon ground nutmeg (Compassion)

- 1/4 cup chopped walnuts (Encouragement)

Instructions:

1. Preheat Oven: Preheat your oven to 350°F (175°C) and line a muffin tin with paper liners, creating a warm and supportive environment.
2. Mix Wet Ingredients: In a large bowl, combine the grated carrots, applesauce, brown sugar, and eggs, mixing well to symbolize empathy, kindness, and care.
3. Combine Dry Ingredients: In another bowl, whisk together the whole wheat flour, baking powder, baking soda, cinnamon, and nutmeg, representing understanding, patience, and balance.
4. Mix Together: Gradually add the dry ingredients to the wet mixture, stirring

until just combined. Fold in the chopped walnuts for encouragement.
5. Bake: Divide the batter evenly among the muffin cups and bake for 20-25 minutes, or until a toothpick inserted into the center comes out clean, emphasizing compassion through a thoughtful and warm treat.
6. Serve: Let the muffins cool before serving, highlighting compassionate care and understanding in every bite.

Recipe 9: Justice Lemon Bars

Ingredients:

- 1 cup all-purpose flour (Fairness)
- 1/2 cup powdered sugar (Equity)
- 1/2 cup butter, softened (Inclusivity)
- 1 cup granulated sugar (Non-discrimination)
- 2 large eggs (Impartiality)

- 1/2 cup fresh lemon juice (Balance)
- 1 tablespoon lemon zest (Transparency)
- 1/4 teaspoon baking powder (Honesty)
- Extra powdered sugar for dusting (Integrity)

Instructions:

1. Preheat Oven: Preheat your oven to 350°F (175°C) and line a baking dish with parchment paper, symbolizing a fair and balanced environment.
2. Prepare Crust: In a bowl, mix the flour, powdered sugar, and softened butter until it forms a crumbly dough, representing fairness and inclusivity. Press the dough evenly into the bottom of the prepared dish.

3. Bake Crust: Bake the crust for 15-20 minutes, or until lightly golden, ensuring a stable foundation of equity.
4. Prepare Filling: In another bowl, whisk together the granulated sugar, eggs, lemon juice, lemon zest, and baking powder until smooth, symbolizing non-discrimination, transparency, and honesty.
5. Bake Filling: Pour the lemon mixture over the baked crust and return to the oven for another 20-25 minutes, or until the filling is set, emphasizing impartiality.
6. Cool and Serve: Let the lemon bars cool completely before dusting with powdered sugar and cutting into squares. Serve, highlighting justice through a balanced and fair dessert.

Recipe 10: Fidelity Pecan Pie Bites

Ingredients:

- 1 cup pecan halves (Commitment)
- 1/2 cup brown sugar (Dependability)
- 1/4 cup butter, melted (Consistency)
- 1/4 cup honey (Trust)
- 1 teaspoon vanilla extract (Loyalty)
- 1/4 teaspoon salt (Faithfulness)
- Mini phyllo shells (Support)

Instructions:

1. Preheat Oven: Preheat your oven to 350°F (175°C) and arrange the mini phyllo shells on a baking sheet, creating a supportive environment.
2. Prepare Filling: In a bowl, mix together the pecan halves, brown sugar, melted butter, honey, vanilla extract, and salt until well combined, symbolizing commitment, dependability, and consistency.
3. Fill Shells: Spoon the pecan mixture into each mini phyllo shell, ensuring

an even distribution to represent trust and loyalty.
4. Bake: Bake for 15-20 minutes, or until the filling is set and the phyllo shells are golden, emphasizing faithfulness and support.
5. Serve: Let the pecan pie bites cool before serving, highlighting fidelity through a dependable and consistent dessert.

Chapter 9: APPETIZERS AND HEALTHY RECIPES

Recipe 1: Empowerment Veggie Dip

Ingredients:

- 1 cup Greek yogurt (Empowerment)
- 1 tablespoon lemon juice (Informed choices)
- 1 teaspoon garlic powder (Respect)

- 1/2 teaspoon onion powder (Transparency)
- 1/4 teaspoon dried dill (Support)
- Salt and pepper to taste (Fairness)
- Assorted fresh vegetables (Carrot sticks, cucumber slices, bell pepper strips) (Health promotion)

Instructions:

1. Prepare Dip: In a bowl, combine Greek yogurt, lemon juice, garlic powder, onion powder, dried dill, salt, and pepper, symbolizing empowerment through informed choices, respect, transparency, and support.
2. Chill: Refrigerate the dip for at least 30 minutes to allow the flavors to meld, emphasizing fairness.

3. Prepare Vegetables: Wash and cut the fresh vegetables into sticks and slices, promoting health promotion.
4. Serve: Arrange the vegetable sticks and slices on a platter around the dip, highlighting the principle of empowerment by allowing individuals to make healthy choices about their snacks.

Recipe 2: Non-maleficence Hummus Platter

Ingredients:

- 1 can chickpeas, drained and rinsed (Minimizing harm)
- 2 cloves garlic, peeled (Preventing risks)
- 2 tablespoons tahini (Safe practices)
- 3 tablespoons lemon juice (Protection)
- 2 tablespoons olive oil (Care)
- Salt and pepper to taste (Safety)

- Assorted fresh vegetables and whole grain pita bread for serving (Supporting well-being)

Instructions:

1. Prepare Hummus: In a food processor, combine the chickpeas, garlic cloves, tahini, lemon juice, olive oil, salt, and pepper, symbolizing the minimization of harm, prevention of risks, and safe practices.
2. Blend: Process until smooth, adding water as needed to achieve the desired consistency, promoting safety.
3. Chill: Transfer the hummus to a serving bowl and refrigerate until ready to serve, ensuring care and protection.
4. Serve: Arrange the hummus bowl on a platter surrounded by fresh vegetables and whole grain pita bread,

highlighting support for well-being through nutritious and wholesome choices.

Recipe 3: Beneficence Quinoa Salad Cups

Ingredients:

- 1 cup cooked quinoa (Health promotion)
- 1/2 cup diced cucumber (Well-being)
- 1/2 cup diced bell pepper (Nourishment)
- 1/4 cup diced red onion (Support)
- 2 tablespoons chopped fresh parsley (Care)
- 2 tablespoons olive oil (Respect for choices)
- 1 tablespoon lemon juice (Empathy)
- Salt and pepper to taste (Positive outcomes)

- Lettuce leaves or endive cups for serving (Comfort)

Instructions:

1. Prepare Salad: In a bowl, combine the cooked quinoa, diced cucumber, diced bell pepper, diced red onion, and chopped fresh parsley, representing health promotion, well-being, nourishment, and care.
2. Dress Salad: Drizzle olive oil and lemon juice over the salad, adding salt and pepper to taste, symbolizing respect for choices, empathy, and positive outcomes.
3. Mix Well: Toss the salad ingredients until evenly coated with the dressing, ensuring support for individuals' well-being.
4. Serve: Spoon the quinoa salad into lettuce leaves or endive cups,

providing comfort and a sense of familiarity in a nutritious and delicious appetizer.

Recipe 4: Justice Stuffed Mushrooms

Ingredients:

- 12 large mushrooms, stems removed and finely chopped (Fairness)
- 1/2 cup breadcrumbs (Equality)
- 1/4 cup grated Parmesan cheese (Equity)
- 2 cloves garlic, minced (Inclusivity)
- 2 tablespoons chopped fresh parsley (Impartiality)
- 2 tablespoons olive oil (Balance)
- Salt and pepper to taste (Fair treatment)
- Cherry tomatoes for garnish (Consideration)

Instructions:

1. Prepare Mushrooms: Preheat your oven to 375°F (190°C) and line a baking sheet with parchment paper. Clean the mushrooms and remove the stems, finely chopping them, symbolizing fairness.
2. Mix Filling: In a bowl, combine the chopped mushroom stems, breadcrumbs, grated Parmesan cheese, minced garlic, chopped fresh parsley, olive oil, salt, and pepper, representing equality, equity, inclusivity, impartiality, and balance.
3. Stuff Mushrooms: Spoon the filling mixture into the mushroom caps, ensuring each is generously filled, promoting fair treatment.
4. Bake: Place the stuffed mushrooms on the prepared baking sheet and bake for 15-20 minutes, or until the mushrooms are golden brown and the

filling is cooked through, demonstrating consideration.

5. Garnish and Serve: Garnish the stuffed mushrooms with cherry tomatoes for an extra burst of flavor and color before serving, highlighting the principle of consideration through thoughtful presentation.

Recipe 5: Confidentiality Cucumber Roll-Ups

Ingredients:

- 1 large cucumber (Privacy)
- 4 ounces cream cheese, softened (Discretion)
- 1 tablespoon chopped fresh dill (Trust)

- 1 tablespoon chopped chives (Security)
- Salt and pepper to taste (Confidential handling)
- Sliced smoked salmon (Confidentiality)

Instructions:

1. Prepare Cucumber: Using a vegetable peeler, slice the cucumber lengthwise into thin strips, representing privacy.
2. Prepare Filling: In a bowl, mix together the softened cream cheese, chopped fresh dill, chopped chives, salt, and pepper, symbolizing discretion, trust, and security.
3. Assemble Roll-Ups: Lay out the cucumber strips and spread a layer of the cream cheese mixture onto each strip. Place a slice of smoked salmon on top of the cream cheese.

4. Roll Up: Carefully roll up each cucumber strip with the cream cheese and smoked salmon inside, ensuring confidential handling.
5. Chill and Serve: Place the cucumber roll-ups on a serving platter and refrigerate until ready to serve, highlighting confidentiality through careful preparation and storage.

These appetizer and healthy recipes further illustrate the principles of medical ethics, demonstrating how ethical conduct can be metaphorically represented through thoughtful, compassionate, and fair preparation of meals.

Recipe 6: Empathy Edamame Salad

Ingredients:

- 2 cups cooked edamame beans (Empathy)
- 1 cup cherry tomatoes, halved (Compassion)
- 1/2 cup diced red onion (Understanding)
- 1/4 cup chopped fresh cilantro (Respect)
- 2 tablespoons lime juice (Support)
- 1 tablespoon olive oil (Care)
- Salt and pepper to taste (Consideration)
- Optional: crumbled feta cheese for garnish (Kindness)

Instructions:

1. Prepare Edamame: If using frozen edamame, cook according to package instructions, then let cool to room temperature, symbolizing empathy.

2. Mix Salad: In a large bowl, combine the cooked edamame beans, cherry tomatoes, diced red onion, and chopped fresh cilantro, representing compassion, understanding, and respect.
3. Dress Salad: Drizzle lime juice and olive oil over the salad, adding salt and pepper to taste, symbolizing support and consideration.
4. Toss Well: Toss the salad ingredients until evenly coated with the dressing, ensuring care.
5. Garnish and Serve: Optionally, garnish the salad with crumbled feta cheese for an extra touch of kindness before serving, highlighting empathy in every bite.

Recipe 7: Integrity Stuffed Bell Peppers

Ingredients:

- 4 large bell peppers, halved and seeds removed (Integrity)
- 1 cup cooked quinoa (Honesty)
- 1 cup black beans, drained and rinsed (Transparency)
- 1 cup corn kernels (Trustworthiness)
- 1 cup diced tomatoes (Fairness)
- 1/2 cup diced red onion (Dependability)
- 1 teaspoon chili powder (Commitment)
- 1/2 teaspoon ground cumin (Consistency)
- Salt and pepper to taste (Balance)
- Optional toppings: avocado slices, chopped cilantro, shredded cheese (Flexibility)

Instructions:

1. Prepare Bell Peppers: Preheat your oven to 375°F (190°C) and line a

baking dish with parchment paper. Place the halved bell peppers in the dish, demonstrating integrity.
2. Mix Filling: In a large bowl, mix together the cooked quinoa, black beans, corn kernels, diced tomatoes, diced red onion, chili powder, ground cumin, salt, and pepper, symbolizing honesty, transparency, trustworthiness, fairness, and dependability.
3. Fill Peppers: Spoon the filling mixture evenly into each bell pepper half, ensuring a commitment to wholesome ingredients.
4. Bake: Cover the baking dish with aluminum foil and bake for 25-30 minutes, or until the peppers are tender, demonstrating consistency and balance.
5. Serve: Optionally, top each stuffed pepper with avocado slices, chopped cilantro, or shredded cheese before

serving, highlighting flexibility in personalizing the dish.

Recipe 8: Non-maleficence Fruit Salsa with Cinnamon Chips

Ingredients:

- 2 apples, diced (Prevention of harm)
- 1 cup diced pineapple (Safety)
- 1 cup diced mango (Minimizing risks)
- 1 cup diced strawberries (Protection)
- 1/4 cup fresh lime juice (Careful consideration)
- 1 tablespoon honey (Balance)
- 1 teaspoon ground cinnamon (Support)
- Whole grain tortillas (Comfort)

Instructions:

1. Prepare Fruit Salsa: In a bowl, combine the diced apples, pineapple, mango, strawberries, fresh lime juice, and honey, symbolizing prevention of harm, safety, minimizing risks, protection, and careful consideration.
2. Chill: Refrigerate the fruit salsa for at least 30 minutes to allow the flavors to meld, emphasizing support and balance.
3. Make Cinnamon Chips: Preheat your oven to 350°F (175°C). Brush whole grain tortillas with a little water and sprinkle with ground cinnamon. Cut into wedges and arrange on a baking sheet.
4. Bake Chips: Bake for 10-12 minutes, or until crispy, promoting comfort.
5. Serve: Serve the fruit salsa with the cinnamon chips for dipping, highlighting non-maleficence through a safe and enjoyable appetizer.

Recipe 9: Justice Greek Stuffed Mushrooms

Ingredients:

- 12 large mushrooms, stems removed and finely chopped (Fairness)
- 1/2 cup cooked quinoa (Equality)
- 1/2 cup crumbled feta cheese (Equity)
- 1/4 cup diced tomatoes (Inclusion)
- 1/4 cup chopped fresh spinach (Non-discrimination)
- 2 tablespoons chopped fresh parsley (Impartiality)
- 2 cloves garlic, minced (Balance)
- Salt and pepper to taste (Fair treatment)

Instructions:

1. Prepare Mushrooms: Preheat your oven to 375°F (190°C) and line a

baking sheet with parchment paper. Clean the mushrooms and remove the stems, finely chopping them, symbolizing fairness.
2. Mix Filling: In a bowl, combine the chopped mushroom stems, cooked quinoa, crumbled feta cheese, diced tomatoes, chopped fresh spinach, chopped fresh parsley, minced garlic, salt, and pepper, representing equality, equity, inclusion, non-discrimination, impartiality, and balance.
3. Fill Mushrooms: Spoon the filling mixture into the mushroom caps, ensuring each is generously filled, promoting fair treatment.
4. Bake: Place the stuffed mushrooms on the prepared baking sheet and bake for 15-20 minutes, or until the mushrooms are tender and the filling is golden brown, emphasizing justice through a balanced and fair dish.

5. Serve: Serve the Greek stuffed mushrooms as a healthy and flavorful appetizer, highlighting the principles of medical ethics in every bite.

Recipe 10: Confidentiality Caprese Skewers

Ingredients:

- Cherry tomatoes (Privacy)
- Fresh mozzarella balls (Discretion)
- Fresh basil leaves (Trust)
- Balsamic glaze (Security)
- Toothpicks or skewers (Confidential handling)

Instructions:

1. Assemble Skewers: Thread a cherry tomato, a fresh mozzarella ball, and a

basil leaf onto each toothpick or skewer, symbolizing privacy, discretion, and trust.
2. Drizzle Glaze: Before serving, drizzle balsamic glaze over the assembled skewers, adding a touch of security.
3. Serve: Arrange the caprese skewers on a platter and serve immediately, emphasizing confidentiality through careful handling and presentation.

30DAY MEAL PLAN

Day 1:

Breakfast: Integrity Granola Bars
Lunch: Respectful Rice Cakes with Hummus and Fresh Vegetables
Dinner: Justice Stuffed Bell Peppers
Snack: Empathy Edamame Salad

Day 2:

Breakfast: Compassionate Caprese Skewers
Lunch: Fidelity Pecan Pie Bites with a Side Salad
Dinner: Beneficence Quinoa Salad Cups
Snack: Non-maleficence Fruit Salsa with Cinnamon Chips

Day 3:

Breakfast: Confidentiality Yogurt Dip with Fresh Fruit
Lunch: Empowerment Veggie Dip with Whole Grain Crackers
Dinner: Non-maleficence Hummus Platter with Whole Wheat Pita Bread
Snack: Justice Greek Stuffed Mushrooms

Day 4:

Breakfast: Beneficence Berry Parfait
Lunch: Integrity Stuffed Mushrooms with a Side Salad
Dinner: Compassionate Carrot Cake Muffins with Steamed Broccoli

Snack: Empathy Apple Slices with Peanut Butter

Day 5:

Breakfast: Justice Lemon Bars
Lunch: Empowerment Veggie Wrap with Hummus
Dinner: Non-maleficence Fruit Salad with Grilled Chicken Breast
Snack: Respectful Raspberry Sorbet

Day 6:

Breakfast: Fidelity Peanut Butter Smoothie
Lunch: Compassionate Cucumber Roll-Ups with Quinoa Salad
Dinner: Beneficence Quinoa Stuffed Bell Peppers
Snack: Confidentiality Caprese Skewers

Day 7:

Breakfast: Integrity Chocolate Avocado Smoothie Bowl
Lunch: Respectful Rice Cakes with Greek Yogurt Dip and Fresh Vegetables
Dinner: Justice Greek Salad with Grilled Shrimp
Snack: Fidelity Pecan Pie Bites

Day 8:

Breakfast: Compassionate Carrot Cake Overnight Oats
Lunch: Integrity Stuffed Mushrooms with Mixed Green Salad
Dinner: Empathy Edamame Salad with Grilled Salmon
Snack: Non-maleficence Hummus Platter with Veggie Sticks

Day 9:

Breakfast: Beneficence Berry Smoothie Bowl
Lunch: Respectful Rice Cakes with Avocado Spread and Tomato Slices

Dinner: Justice Greek Stuffed Bell Peppers with Quinoa Salad
Snack: Fidelity Peanut Butter Energy Bites

Day 10:

Breakfast: Empowerment Veggie Omelette with Whole Wheat Toast
Lunch: Confidentiality Caprese Salad with Balsamic Glaze
Dinner: Compassionate Quinoa-Stuffed Zucchini Boats
Snack: Respectful Raspberry Sorbet

Day 11:

Breakfast: Non-maleficence Fruit Salad with Greek Yogurt
Lunch: Justice Mediterranean Wrap with Hummus
Dinner: Integrity Lentil and Vegetable Soup with Whole Grain Bread
Snack: Empathy Apple Slices with Almond Butter

Day 12:

Breakfast: Fidelity Overnight Chia Seed Pudding with Fresh Berries
Lunch: Beneficence Quinoa Salad Cups with Grilled Chicken Strips
Dinner: Respectful Baked Salmon with Roasted Vegetables
Snack: Confidentiality Cucumber Roll-Ups with Cream Cheese

Day 13:

Breakfast: Compassionate Banana Walnut Muffins
Lunch: Empowerment Veggie Stir-Fry with Tofu
Dinner: Non-maleficence Hummus Platter with Whole Grain Crackers
Snack: Justice Greek Yogurt with Honey and Mixed Nuts

Day 14:

Breakfast: Integrity Granola with Greek Yogurt and Fresh Fruit
Lunch: Respectful Rice Cakes with Avocado and Tomato Slices
Dinner: Beneficence Quinoa-Stuffed Peppers with Grilled Shrimp
Snack: Fidelity Peanut Butter Smoothie

Day 15:

Breakfast: Compassionate Carrot Cake Overnight Oats
Lunch: Integrity Stuffed Mushrooms with Mixed Green Salad
Dinner: Empathy Edamame Salad with Grilled Salmon
Snack: Non-maleficence Hummus Platter

with Veggie Sticks

Day 16:

Breakfast: Beneficence Berry Smoothie Bowl
Lunch: Respectful Rice Cakes with Avocado Spread and Tomato Slices

Dinner: Justice Greek Stuffed Bell Peppers with Quinoa Salad
Snack: Fidelity Peanut Butter Energy Bites

Day 17:

Breakfast: Empowerment Veggie Omelette with Whole Wheat Toast
Lunch: Confidentiality Caprese Salad with Balsamic Glaze
Dinner: Compassionate Quinoa-Stuffed Zucchini Boats
Snack: Respectful Raspberry Sorbet

Day 18:

Breakfast: Non-maleficence Fruit Salad with Greek Yogurt
Lunch: Justice Mediterranean Wrap with Hummus
Dinner: Integrity Lentil and Vegetable Soup with Whole Grain Bread
Snack: Empathy Apple Slices with Almond Butter

Day 19:

Breakfast: Fidelity Overnight Chia Seed Pudding with Fresh Berries
Lunch: Beneficence Quinoa Salad Cups with Grilled Chicken Strips
Dinner: Respectful Baked Salmon with Roasted Vegetables
Snack: Confidentiality Cucumber Roll-Ups with Cream Cheese

Day 20:

Breakfast: Compassionate Banana Walnut Muffins
Lunch: Empowerment Veggie Stir-Fry with Tofu
Dinner: Non-maleficence Hummus Platter with Whole Grain Crackers
Snack: Justice Greek Yogurt with Honey and Mixed Nuts

Day 21:

Breakfast: Integrity Granola with Greek Yogurt and Fresh Fruit
Lunch: Respectful Rice Cakes with Avocado and Tomato Slices
Dinner: Beneficence Quinoa-Stuffed Peppers with Grilled Shrimp
Snack: Fidelity Peanut Butter Smoothie

Day 22:

Breakfast: Compassionate Carrot Cake Overnight Oats
Lunch: Integrity Stuffed Mushrooms with Mixed Green Salad
Dinner: Empathy Edamame Salad with Grilled Salmon
Snack: Non-maleficence Hummus Platter

with Veggie Sticks

Day 23:

Breakfast: Beneficence Berry Smoothie Bowl
Lunch: Respectful Rice Cakes with Avocado Spread and Tomato Slices

Dinner: Justice Greek Stuffed Bell Peppers with Quinoa Salad
Snack: Fidelity Peanut Butter Energy Bites

Day 24:

Breakfast: Empowerment Veggie Omelette with Whole Wheat Toast
Lunch: Confidentiality Caprese Salad with Balsamic Glaze
Dinner: Compassionate Quinoa-Stuffed Zucchini Boats
Snack: Respectful Raspberry Sorbet

Day 25:

Breakfast: Non-maleficence Fruit Salad with Greek Yogurt
Lunch: Justice Mediterranean Wrap with Hummus
Dinner: Integrity Lentil and Vegetable Soup with Whole Grain Bread
Snack: Empathy Apple Slices with Almond Butter

Day 26:

Breakfast: Fidelity Overnight Chia Seed Pudding with Fresh Berries
Lunch: Beneficence Quinoa Salad Cups with Grilled Chicken Strips
Dinner: Respectful Baked Salmon with Roasted Vegetables
Snack: Confidentiality Cucumber Roll-Ups with Cream Cheese

Day 27:

Breakfast: Compassionate Banana Walnut Muffins
Lunch: Empowerment Veggie Stir-Fry with Tofu
Dinner: Non-maleficence Hummus Platter with Whole Grain Crackers
Snack: Justice Greek Yogurt with Honey and Mixed Nuts

Day 28:

Breakfast: Integrity Granola with Greek Yogurt and Fresh Fruit
Lunch: Respectful Rice Cakes with Avocado and Tomato Slices
Dinner: Beneficence Quinoa-Stuffed Peppers with Grilled Shrimp
Snack: Fidelity Peanut Butter Smoothie

Day 29:

Breakfast: Compassionate Carrot Cake Overnight Oats
Lunch: Integrity Stuffed Mushrooms with Mixed Green Salad
Dinner: Empathy Edamame Salad with Grilled Salmon
Snack: Non-maleficence Hummus Platter with Veggie Sticks

Day 30:

Breakfast: Beneficence Berry Smoothie Bowl
Lunch: Respectful Rice Cakes with Avocado Spread and Tomato Slices

Dinner: Justice Greek Stuffed Bell Peppers with Quinoa Salad
Snack: Fidelity Peanut Butter Energy Bites

CONCLUSION

"Nourishing the Body, Nurturing the Soul: A Recipe for Ethical Wellness

In the pursuit of health and wellness, we often forget that food is not just fuel, but a fundamental aspect of our humanity. The Medical Ethics Cookbook is more than just a collection of recipes - it's a testament to the power of nutrition to heal, connect, and inspire.

Within these pages, you'll discover:

Delicious, easy-to-make recipes that prioritize whole, nutritious ingredients
Inspiring stories of healthcare professionals who embody the principles of medical ethics

Practical tips for navigating the complex landscape of healthcare and nutrition

This cookbook is a call to action, inviting you to embrace the interconnectedness of food, health, and ethics. By nourishing our bodies and honoring the values of medical ethics, we can create a world where everyone has the opportunity to thrive.

Join the movement. Savor the flavor. Nourish your soul. Get your copy of the Medical Ethics Cookbook today!"

THE END

www.ingramcontent.com/pod-product-compliance
Lightning Source LLC
Chambersburg PA
CBHW071209240526
45470CB00018B/1652